Relapsing Remitting
Multiple Sclerosis

Relapsing Remitting Multiple Sclerosis

HOW TO COPE WITH MULTIPLE SCLEROSIS

La Tasha Shelton

To order additional copies of this book, contact:
Xlibris LLC
1-888-795-4274
www.Xlibris.com
Orders@Xlibris.com
620596

Contents

Biography

My name is La Tasha Rochelle Shelton. I was born to Lizzie and Tommy Shelton in Little Rock, Arkansas. I am the older of two children. I have a younger sister named Renetta Shelton and two half-brothers whom my father had in previous relationships. My childhood was not that great. My dad was a drinker, smoker, abused my mom as well as cheated on her for years until me and my sister had said enough was enough. My mom was a workaholic who made sure that me and my sister was well taken care of. My mom depended on me too much when I was younger. She required me to look after my sister, and if she does something wrong, I was the one to get punished for it because I was the oldest and should have prevented her for doing wrong. I was raised in a strict household were me and my sister wasn't allowed to do anything but play in the front yard. We were never allowed to go over our friends' houses, but they were allowed to come over ours. I guess being raised in a strict home made me do things my mom didn't approve of let along found out about. I did a lot of sneaky things as a kid. What child you know doesn't? When my mom divorced my dad, we moved into Hemlock Courts (the projects) when I was fourteen years old and my dad abandoned us. I attended Leach Chapel CME church in North Little Rock, Arkansas was Pastor Clinton L. Washington presided at the time. RIP. I was baptized at the age of fourteen. Pastor Washington was the guy who I looked up to as a father figure. He and his wife took me under their wing and treated me like their own. When he died from cancer, it hurted me so bad because he was like a father that I never had. I still miss him till this day. Now that he is gone, who was going to step up to the plate now, when my biological father wasn't around for me? I now attend Mount Pisgah Baptist Church under the leadership of Pastor Craig B. Collier in Jacksonville, Arkansas. When I was seventeen, we moved into another project called Windermere Courts in Little Rock, Arkansas. Though I was having family issues, I still remained an honor student all the way to the eleventh grade. In my last year of high school, we moved into a house, and attended The Little Rock Central High school in Little Rock, Arkansas. There I graduated with a 2.4 G.P.A. That was a great drop from having a 3.5 G.P.A. when I attended North Little Rock High School West Campus in North Little Rock, Arkansas. It was not until I graduated High school was when my dad decided to show up. I was mad at my dad for years because he left us to struggle with our mom all because she had divorced him. I learned to forgive and give my dad a second chance to make amends. He was always there when I graduated from college, but emotionally not there for me when I needed to understand how a man was to treat a woman because he wasn't a good man to my mother. So, I thought I could find love and a father figure in the guys I've dated. I was very wrong. I had friends who I have grown up with find spouses that made them very happy. I had never been married; I had three sons out of wedlock with men who were not right for me. I am a single mother without the help of their fathers. I am an overcomer simply because I did not let my disappointments in life deter me from achieving my goals in life. I also became very rebellious with my mom because I thought she was too hard on me as a child and loved my sister more than me. I never really gotten over the way she had treated me when I was young. Still to this day, I don't have a good relationship with her. I blamed her for everything that went wrong in my life and she blames me as well. I have achieved a lot in life, and my mom was there, but she did not say how happy she was for me to finish college and doing something with my life. I felt like she hated to call me her daughter because of the hell I put her through when I was growing up. I believed she loved my sister more than me because of the way she would do things and go places with her, but never with me. She told me that she did not do things with me because I told her when I was a teenager that I hated her. Still to this day, she still does it. She is only friendly with me when she wants me to do something for her. At times, I find myself trying to please her more than pleasing myself. I look for her approval of the guys I choose to be with and I'm thirty two years old. I wonder why I am not married. She always finds a way to run the guys I date off. I feel she wants me to stay single like her for the rest of my life. That is not going to happen to me! She wants to control my life and I am not going to allow it to happen anymore. From this day forward, I am choosing me! I will not allow anyone to hurt me anymore. I am going to live for me and my children. I want the best for me. I have for too long been caring what others think of me. Not anymore. I am going to do what God and myself is set out too, and that is go back to college and finish up my education and nursing degree and find a job that will allow me to show my skills and talents for all the world to see. Look out world, La Tasha is coming through. You either have to live life or let life control you. Either way, you have to make a decision on the path you want to take. To those people who said I couldn't do it, May God have mercy on you! I have no regrets in the choices I have made in life, and you shouldn't either. I encourage you to move on with what God has given you and do all you can to ensure you have a secure future set up for yourself and your kids. Don't worry about the haters, just keep your eyes on GOD, who is always there to guide you down that path he wants you take.

Finding out that you have Multiple Sclerosis

One day I was sitting in my living room watching television when I had this tingling sensation in my legs that was so uncomfortable that I did not know what was wrong with me. I started to cry. I wanted to know what was going on with me, so I went to the emergency room only to find out that the doctors did not know what was wrong with me. So I went on with my daily life which consisted of going to college, working, and taking care of three sons on my own with the help of my mom and sister of course. The next day, I went to work doing what I always do, when my hands went numb and the muscles went out of control that it caused me severe pain, and I could not hold or pick up anything without dropping it. I did not want to take the chance of going back to the emergency room and have the doctors tell me that they could not find anything wrong with me again, so I ignored the second symptom. This was a big mistake. I was cleaning one day, matter of fact it was a couple of days after my birthday that my whole right side of my body went completely numb. I had no feeling or could I feel any pain on my right side. This prompted me to go back to the emergency room a second time. This time, I told the doctors what was going on and they decided to call a neurologist in to see me. In the back of my mind, I was wondering what in the world would they want to call in a neurologist for. The neurologist ran a series of tests to see what was going on. The neurologist and his team of student doctors came into my room only to tell me that what I was going through was one of two autoimmune diseases such as Lupus and Multiple Sclerosis. The neurologist ran more tests only to discover that I have Relapsing Remitting Multiple Sclerosis. He told me that he had to get me well for the sake of my three sons. At the time, I did not know what Multiple Sclerosis was because there was no one in my family who had this type of illness. I was wondering how I am supposed to be able to take care of my sons when I became sick. I was a single mother who wanted to get married, live a long healthy life so I am able to see my sons grow up and become successful citizens in society. How was I supposed to achieve this now that I have M.S.? I thought my world was shattered and there was nothing I could do to change it? I believe in GOD, and I started to question my existence when I became sick. I tried to go on with my daily life, but it became hard because I was in denial of my illness. I tried to block out the idea of even having M.S. at all. Every time I tried, my body reminded me that M.S. was there and I just couldn't ignore it. My neurologist had prescribed me a medicine called Copaxone injections that I have to take every day to prevent a major relapse from happening. When I first started the injections, I was very hesitant at first, because I hated needles, but I knew that if I wanted to get well, I must take these injections. I also knew I had three sons who needed me, and I realized that I needed to do whatever I needed to do to stay healthy and live a healthy lifestyle for the sake of my children. Having M.S. had changed the way I look at life. I found myself even more depressed than I initially was because I became angry at the fact that I had this autoimmune disease that was incurable, and that I felt alone and did not know who to talk to, so I shut everybody out and decided that I was not going to deal with this illness at all. I was wrong; I found out that if I talked about it, I would feel better. That did not work for me at all. I became very emotional and very angry for having to deal with this illness on a daily basis. Why should I deal with something that I feel should not be happening to me? I thought God was punishing me for something I did in my past. I was trying to come up with ways as to why I had M.S. and I could not find anything. Had I live my life so bad that I have now begun to pay the price for my past mistakes? These were questions I was asking myself. I could not talk to my mom or sister about my feelings because they did not understand why I was having these emotional break downs and taking my frustrations out on them. There was a point when I thought everybody was my enemy. Nobody wanted to come around me because of my anger issues. I was pushing my kids away and treating them like they were my enemy and that was not right. So I decided to channel all my energy by battling my problems inwardly and that was the wrong thing to do as well. I even contemplated suicide thinking if I could take myself out the picture the better the world would be. M.S. became the worst in my life and I did not know what to do to deal or live with an illness that could be the beginning or the end of my life. So I discovered prayer. I felt that if I focused my mind on a higher power, the less my frustrations with my illness would be. I realize that I had put GOD on the back burner and myself first and that was not what GOD intended me to do. He has proven himself more and more to me in my life than I realized. If GOD had not stepped in like he did, I would not have known where I would be this day. Writing this book is very important to me because it allows me to show the real me and to let the world know that having M.S. doesn't mean the end of your life, but just the beginning of a new you in GOD and the people around you. Telling you my life story allows me to heal and give you the hope that if you turn a negative situation into a positive one, you can live a life that is full of love, peace, and a excitement that you can prove to yourself and anyone out there that you can survive! I hope this book is an encouraging one to anyone who not only goes through an illness, but can overcome it if they fight. You cannot give up, you must fight; that is the only way you can defeat the enemy. M.S. does not have to end your life or put it on hold. You must take back your life and do what you have to do to overcome this disease. Don't let the Devil win, because Victory is yours in Christ Jesus and you are an overcomer.

What is Relapsing Remitting Multiple Sclerosis?

Relapsing Remitting Multiple Sclerosis is often characterized by relapses (exacerbation) followed by periods of remission in which the person fully or partially recovers from the deficits acquired during relapse. Relapse can last for days, weeks, or months and recovery can be slow and gradual or instantaneous. You develop RRMS between the age of 20 and 30 years of age. During relapses, myelin, a protective insulating sheath around the nerve fibers (neurons) in the white matter regions of the CNS (Central Nervous System), is damaged in an inflammatory response by the body's own immune system. This causes a wide variety of neurological symptoms that vary depending on which areas of the CNS are damaged. After a relapse, the inflammatory response dies down and a special type of glial cell in the CNS (called an oligodendrocyte) sponsors demyelination-a process where the myelin sheath around the axon is repaired. It is this demyelination that is responsible for the remission. Approximately 50% of patients with Relapsing Remitting Multiple Sclerosis convert to Secondary Progressive Multiple Sclerosis (SPMS) within ten years of disease onset. After thirty years this figure rises to 90%.

Living with Relapsing Remitting Multiple Sclerosis

Living with Relapsing Remitting Multiple Sclerosis depends on how well you deal with the flare ups and debilating malfunctions it entails. As for me, I have experience vision changes, uncontrollable muscle movements, and heaviness in my legs, slurred speech, and nerve damage in my face. I have also had fallen and bump into walls and furniture due to me not being able to balance myself well. Having RRMS had not caused me to have a major relapse or to become hospitalized. I must on the other hand take daily injections to prevent a major relapse from occurring. Living with RRMS had allowed me to appreciate life and those things we often take for granted. There are times I wish I could be healthy, but I know that is impossible to achieve. When I became diagnosed with RRMS, I became very depressed and so heavy burdened that I wanted to end it all. I did not want to put my mom and children, through the ups and downs of this illness. I did not want anyone to have to take care of me for the rest of my life. I am supposed to take care of my mom when she reaches old age, not her having to take care of me. I am only thirty two years old; why am I stricken with a disease that could very much erase me from society and that of my true family and friends. Having Relapsing Remitting Multiple Sclerosis has really changed my life. I am battling mentally with this illness every single day, and I don't know how to allow myself to get back to me so to speak. I am constantly depressed and lost all hope and faith to defeating this disease. What am I to do? I can't talk to my family because they do not understand and I can't even find the strength to pray to GOD whom I have a good relationship with. It seems like I have given up on the life I once had. I have tried to involve myself in activities that could give me happiness, but I find myself smiling on the outside, but depressed on the inside. I find myself pleasing other people and not myself. I don't want to burden anyone with my problems because I don't want anyone to judge me. I am in need of a positive influence not a negative one. I don't want to pay a therapist to tell me what I already know about myself. I am so overwhelmed to the point that I want to crawl in a hole and to never be seen again. RRMS had changed me so much mentally and physically that I don't know how else to be to myself and to other people who I am in contact with every day. I am not writing this book to put anyone down, I am writing this book to prove to anyone who is battling any illness to find within you the inner strength to continue to live life to the fullest. I want this book to give anyone that is sick the encouragement to want to live life like you use to. I cannot speak for everyone, but I can speak about myself and encourage myself in living with an illness that will not disappear to fight this illness. With all that, I am much stronger than I allow myself to believe. With all that is going on, I for one should be strong. I am strong for everyone else, and I am the one who my mom depend on to succeed. When I became sick, my world changed. Now it is up to me to find ways to cope with this illness. Oh what a day it will be when I learn and am able to testify to others that you might not beat this illness, but you can give it your all in fighting this illness if you do not give up. Don't allow yourself to become defeated; you continue to fight for the life you are destined to have. Do what is necessary to live life to the fullest with no regrets; but with progress!

Journal letters

7/6/2012

Sometimes I feel like I don't deserve to live. M.S. has ruined my life. Why do I have this illness? Why me Lord, why am I the one who have to get sick? I have three sons who I have to live for and who needs me. What have I done to deserve this? Am I being punished for my past mistakes or am I the one you chose to make an example out of for those who need to be drawn closer to you? Lord helps me to understand. I am at a lost here. I need you more now than I ever did before. Can you please help me to cope with an illness that is incurable? I will do whatever you need me to do. You want me to serve you more, I will; you need me to pray more, I will; you need me to tithe more I will. I will do whatever you need me to do to just be healed from this illness. I want to be a teacher. I cannot be a teacher if I can't stand for long periods of time. My memory is not that great. I need to remember the important things. How can I be a teacher if my memories of the lessons to be taught are not there? Is there any way for you to deliver me out of this ailment? I need you now, and I know only you can help me to defeat this disease we call M.S.

7/10/2012

Today was not a good day. I woke up with this funny feeling in my head. I am not a 100% today. I don't know where my strength is going to come from. I have so much to do and no strength or energy to accomplished the tasks I have today. Lord gives me strength to do these tasks and spend time with my children. They need me, and I need you to allow me this opportunity to complete these tasks that is very demanding of me to complete. In Jesus name, I pray. Amen.

I decided to start writing journal letters to help me to express my feelings on a daily basis. When I write my true feelings down, my stress level becomes less and less relevant to what I am dealing with, and I begin the healing process; Though I just begun writing my thoughts down, I hope what you read relates to what you are dealing with and gives you a sense of hope to want to live your life as you once did. Know that you are not alone and that someone out there is going through what you are going through and that you just need to connect with someone that can help you to cope and encourage you to continue to fight and not to give up on yourself or life. My life with RRMS is not a good pill to swallow when you finally realize you have a disease that is incurable and only going to get worst as the years goes by. I have yet to see anyone discuss what it feels like to have an illness such as this that going to impact your whole life. It would be nice for people to walk in your shoes to see the many emotional changes RRMS has caused the people who have it. It would be nice to feel good about defeating this illness without all the criticisms of others who do not have a clue about what goes on in the lives or minds of people who have to live with this particular disease. It is easy for an outsider to say 'Oh you will get through it' or have faith in GOD, if you have never been sick before. I wish there was enough information out there or people or doctors would give seminars on Multiple Sclerosis to the world so that people who struggle with this illness would not be treated different or written off just because you are sick. I am not asking for pity, I'm asking for the right to be treated fairly by people who do not have a clue as to what I am going through. Yes RRMS is debilitating, but we do not expect to be treated like we are already. Allow

Us live life as normal as possible. I am telling my story and hope whoever reads it can help those who need the encouragement to fight. Our journey is not over; it's just beginning!

7/11/2012

Today I am in pain. I woke up very sore, and I am not that motivated at all. But I have forced my way to write what was on my mind. Though I am in pain, I am still able to record my feelings here. I find that recording my feelings day to day helps me and relieves some of the stress I am dealing with that I am not able in share with anyone else.

8/6/2012

Today is not a good day. I am in pain again, but this time it's in my left thigh and leg. It seems as if my M.S. is affecting different parts of my body so much so that I don't know what to do about it. I keep on moving around in hopes that the pain would ease. I take Ibuprofen to stop the pain and it works for a while, but the pain comes back. I pray all the time mentally because I just can't find the strength to get on my knees. I feel as if I could have a normal life some days, and other days I am severely depressed and don't know how I am going to get through each day without feeling the world is caving in on me. My children know that I am sick but don't understand why their mom is mean, angry, and don't have the energy to play with them like I use to do. They shower me with hugs and kisses to make me smile, and it works. I look in their faces and see their love they have for me and try to fight harder each day to spend the time and find the energy to do what they want to do.

8/21/2012

Today is a fair day. I am not in pain, but I am still battling this illness mentally. Before I found out I had RRMS, I had a lot of Depression issues.

It was a very dark place in my life that I did not know how to come out of. I could not talk to anyone and I was very sad, and I thought my life was over. Nobody wants to feel like they don't mean anything to anyone at any given moment. But at the time, I was feeling exile from my family and did not know how to deal with it all. I can't explain how I got through my darkest hour, but I do know who brought me out. Religion plays a big part in my life and it helps me to get through the most difficult days in my life. I am still trying to find my purpose in life. When I do, I know I could do some great things for myself, my family, and my community.

RRMS have changed my life so much that I myself can't really understand the many flare ups in my body that hinders me from the life I am use to living. I find myself encouraging myself when everything around me seem to be falling to pieces. I have not given up on my life at all. I am fighting each and every day for the sake of my kids and myself.

What's Next?

RRMS has taught me to realize how not to take life, and my body for granted. Because once you do, it can be taken away in a blink of an eye. I do not know what the future holds for me with this illness, but I know that I am not going to give up the fight to live my life as God wants me to live it and that is in him. RRMS has allowed me to appreciate what I have and cherish it; for what it's worth, if it had not been for this illness, I'd probably be living life with risks and not thinking about the consequences I would have to face along the way. RRMS does not mean I have to stop living, it means I just have to continue on this journey called life no matter what this illness entails. I must push forward and not let anything get in the way. RRMS has and always will be a major part of my life. I am getting much better in accepting this disease by knowing my limits and recognizing that RRMS does not have to end my life but embrace it. I will endure to the end! Life is a challenge when you have to focus on an illness that very well could make your future and that of your children. My encouragement to everyone who is battling Multiple Sclerosis is to never stop fighting. You have to change the way you think. How you think about your illness can play a part in how well you deal with it. My goal in life is to beat Multiple Sclerosis and not it beat me. You have to have an inner champion within you that will not let you settle for what the doctors, family, or people in the community dictate how you should battle this disease. It is not over! It's the beginning to where God has destined you to be. You are a testimony to yourself and to those who looks to the fighter within you. You do what you have to do to live a productive life. Life is much sweeter if you put more effort into getting better whether than worrying what people are going to say about you. I am willing to fight with all my might to live for my children. My children are what motivate me to keep on living. Whatever you are battling with whether it is your job, family, friends, let it go and take care of you! If you let these affect your ability to get better, it only will make things worse than they already are. You don't need stress. Multiple Sclerosis is stress enough. Don't let what people say affect your life. If you don't have a good support system, I suggest you get one. Having a good support system will give you the strength to move forward in what you want to do without limitations. My support system is my mom and sister. They helps me a lot with my children, allows me to get away when I need to, and gives me love when I am depressed or not feeling myself. They allow me to keep on moving and that if I need them, they will always be there. I thank God for allowing me to have a good support system. God is my top support system! He never left me or forsake me. He's there when I need him and he always takes care of me. I know I talk a lot about God, but he is the one who allowed be to be able to be stricken with a disease and still have the ability of my limbs, and the ability to see, and speak. Why not give him praise. He has gotten me through the worst of days and I am very grateful. I find comfort and peace in him. Try him for yourself. I telling you am good, but you have to experience him for yourself. He gotten me over many health problems, and I believe he will get me over this. Multiple Sclerosis is indeed another hurdle I must get over, but I believe I can do all things in Christ who strengthens me (Philippians 4:13). Multiple Sclerosis may be a health threat, but it is not a hindrance in my life. It should be a hindrance in yours either. Set a goal as to what you going to do to make your life as efficient so that you can live a happy life. Life is fulfilling if you eliminate some of the stresses. I know what I say is easier said than done, but if you apply yourself, and focus on getting better and living a fulfilling life in which you are happy, then you can defeat this illness. Remember: You have to change your mind set in order to better deal with your illness. If you have a positive mindset the better you are able to accept it. Again, change your mindset and make decisions on how you live your life. The better you're able to deal with Multiple Sclerosis head-on, the better you are able to cope with it. It's not going to be easy; you have to take one day at a time to fully decide how you are going to deal with this illness. Once you have made up in your mind that you are going to tackle this illness head-on the better your life becomes. Do whatever is necessary to enjoy life to the fullest capacity. With the help of your support system, you can get the strength to accomplish any goals you had set for your life. Don't let this illness choose the life you ought to live, you choose how you want to live. Smile, you can do it! Encourage yourself daily, or write down encouraging words that gives you the motivation to move forward in life. Become the person you want to be, not the person people want you to be.

I am not saying I'm perfect, It took me a long time to realized I had to make a decision in my life that is going to change my life for the better. In order for me to move forward in life, I had to remove some people out my life that do not have my best interest at heart. I am not at my best every day, but I do realize who gives me the strength when I am at my lowest. Nobody in this world could make me as happy as having the faith in God to guide me on a path where I am walking in the light. Having that faith in God gives me hope in beating this disease. My future looks brighter every year. I see what God has done and still is doing in my life and that of my family. I encourage anyone who reads this book to try Him before you doubt him. Give him a chance to do what he is set out to do before you give up on him. I know you ask the question WHY. I been there and still am where you are now. I believe and have the faith in him enough to trust him with my whole heart and soul. Before you give up on him, try him and watch him change your situation. Yes you may be having a lot of health problems, but be content and have patience. He will give you joy, and there is power in Jesus name if you just call on him.

This gets me through every day I wake up. I have to encourage myself to do the things I'm not feeling well to do at times. I keep telling myself that it is not over; it's only the beginning for me and everyone else who is fighting a disease on a daily basis. I just say keep your head up, and keep on fighting. It will get better by and by. Trust in yourself to do what you have to do to be here for your children. They need you more than you know. Keep fighting for them. If nothing else motivates you, your children should be the one who gives you the strength and motivation to continue to fight this battle.

Treatment

Treating Relapsing Remitting Multiple Sclerosis is a hard task for anyone who is dealing with this illness has to cope with. I am on a very mild dose of Copaxone injections that I must take every single day. To be honest, I don't like this drug simply because it causes lumps, indentations, and it burns a lot. You would think that after battling with this disease for four years the burning would stop, but it has not. So, I suggest to all of you who are battling with this illness to try different medicines to see which one is the right one for you, and not settle for just one that the doctor prescribes. You have to do what you feel would accommodate your body not what goes against it. Treating your Multiple Sclerosis may be hard to commit to, but I guarantee that if you stay on a regular treatment plan, the lesser the relapses. I have been on copaxone for four years now, I have had two more spots showed up in my brain, now my doctors is debating on whether or not they should give me a stronger treatment to prevent further spots or keep me on the same dose. This concerns me a lot, because I have three sons who need me. I am going to do whatever is necessary to ensure that I be around for my sons. I must be strong enough to want to better my health for myself. You can do it too. You have to want to get better, and you have to do whatever it takes to ensure you be around for those who need you the most. There have to be a fighter in you to want to defeat this illness no matter the cost. Do what you have to do, to be here; you do have a life to live as everyone else. Remember the good years before Multiple Sclerosis; don't let the years pass you by because of an illness. Step out on faith; let God lead you to your destiny, and not you. You cannot predict the future or what your life supposed to be. Live for right now, because tomorrow is not promised. You want to know how I became so positive. I realized that I cannot dread on an illness I cannot get rid of. It took me a long time to get to this point in my life. It was a time that I could not bring up the word Multiple Sclerosis without crying, or even talk about it to anyone. I am not completely over it still, though I am writing it down in this book. I have learn to get back into Gods word, pray consistently, and put all my trust in God to know that HE will take care of it. Now, I am speaking boldly to members of my church and people who feel they have no hope in getting better. I feel that if I could be a testimony to someone who is sick and don't know who to turn to, why not me. I have a wonderful testimony for those who think that God cannot bring them out of their situation. You are looking at a woman who not only battle Multiple Sclerosis, but almost had Cervical Cancer, and who almost did not wake up from surgery during gall bladder removal, I am a witness to what God can do for the sick. I am not telling you what I heard; I am telling you what I know. I look at the world much different than before. I am focus on what I can give back to the world, instead of what I can take from it. That is why it is so important for you to be an encouragement to yourself; if you cannot encourage yourself, who is going to do it? You cannot wait on the world to do it; it will let you down every time. So, that is why you have to do it for yourself; you cannot wait on anyone else to do it, you have to do it. Once you have made up in your mind that you are going to live for you and nobody else, the journey of your life begins. You have to want to change in order for a change to come. The road is not gone be easy, but you have to want to get through the challenges in order to heal. That is why I look up to Robin Roberts so much; during her battle with cancer, she is not letting it defeat her. She is fighting this illness with a smile on her face. Yes she have some down days, but she do not let it stop her from accomplishing what God has set out for her to do. You have to do the same. Don't let your illness stop you from living life. Live life as God wants you to live it; and that is with a smile on your face, pep in your step, and a will to do whatever it takes to ensure that everyone that is battling this disease have a hope that one day they will find a cure. If they don't then you be an encouragement for somebody else. Move forward in your destiny! Everyone has a life to live and a short time to live it. Everyone has to die one day; Leave a legacy behind for those who knew you, so that your spirit lives on in your family. This may be easier said than done, but it can be accomplish is you are willing to change your mindset. Your mindset is what can make or break you; that is why you must put positive things into your mind. Your mind is the biggest thing that could ruin or make your life as successful as you choose it to be. Once you remove the negative things and replace them with positive, the more or stronger you can be in coping with your illness.

Moving Forward

Now that you have all the necessary tools to deal with your illness, now it is time to move forward to what lies ahead of you. Moving Forward means to let go of all that was holding you back from living the life you once lived before. You do this by completing what you have started. Like me, I started writing a book about my life, and now am completing it for all to read. When you found out you had Relapsing Remitting Multiple Sclerosis, didn't it seem that your life was put on hold because you had to battle a disease that was out of your control? Don't feel bad, I felt the same way. When I became sick, I thought everything I was trying to accomplish in life was untouchable because I was sick. It seems like everything has slowed down to a point that I was never going to reach it. My life seem to slow from its fast pace, to a more slow, frustrated pace that I was not comfortable with. All of a sudden, my focus was gone, writing ability has changed, eyes were not seeing things like they use to, and speech was becoming more of a challenge. All this has happen to me all at once, and I did not know how to cope with it all. I became depressed, stressed out, frustrated and very angry because my life has changed and there was nothing I could do about it. Sounds familiar? I've been here, and still where you are now. So, don't feel bad, or out of place. I come to realized that as long as I was stressing about what my life could have been without Multiple Sclerosis I wouldn't been able to help others get through theirs. That is why I've made up in my mind that I was not going to let my illness destroy me, and you should not either. I've decided to move forward with the life I have now, and not dread on what it could have been. I've decided to live life despite what limitations I have. I had figured that if I focus on what today holds for me, and not what tomorrow will bring, the better I will be in the eyes of those who looks up to me. I cannot change the future or the past, so why am I stressing about it. Life is too short to be worrying about things that are out of our control. That's why you should turn your negative thoughts in positive ones and let no one deter you from your hopes and dreams. I had never thought that I was going to write a book about my life with Multiple Sclerosis and all the stresses it brings. I never thought I would ever be at the point to where I could encourage others to be strong and not let their illness define who they are. My challenge to you is, to not let people, family, friends, or coworkers talk negative about your illness to you. You must be strong enough to turn what they say to you into something positive. Show them that your illness does not define who you are, it just make you an overcomer. Use your obstacle as a testimony to your friends, family, church members, and coworkers. Don't let your illness stop you from achieving your goals; move forward and show those who was against you that you are truly an overcomer and an achiever.

Be Grateful

The final step in knowing that you are moving forward is to know that you are grateful for the life and the support system you have. To have the both of these is an accomplishment in itself. You can't move forward with life if you don't have a strong system behind you encouraging you to live the life you was destined to live. Grateful means being appreciative of the benefits being received; to me that means that you are a grateful person when you are thankful for everything everybody has done for you throughout your life. I believe that if you give back to those who have helped you along the way, the more blessed you become. You cannot move forward if you do not appreciate the ones who made your life as successful it is today. I want to take the time to thank my mom for pushing me into becoming that successful woman I am today. I know that if she hadn't push me, I probably be dead, or in jail. My mom is the person I gave the most hell throughout my life, because my father wasn't in the picture as much as she was. I want to let her know that I do really love her, and that when push comes to shove, she is always there when I needed her the most or when I was in my darkest hour. There is no one in this world that could ever replace my mother. You only get one mother in this lifetime; why not cherish her why she is still living. Because when she is gone, there is nothing you can do about it. Give her flowers why she is yet alive. My mom has been there for me when everyone turns their back on me. She took a lot of slack from me, especially when I became sick, angry, and frustrated. She took it all and never left me. Who do you know would do that for you? I know no one that could; so I advise you to fix the relationship with your family right now, because you will never find another family who would stick closer to you than family or Jesus Christ. I live for family, and I would never ever disrespect them as I did in the past ever again. I am very grateful for everything in life and I might regret some mistakes I have made, but I do not punish myself for them. I just live life each day as if it was my last day on this earth. I am enjoying life to the fullest with no regrets. Moving forward to what God has for me, and not letting anyone take away from it to better their life. Help others, and it will be returned unto you. Take away from it, and Karma will show up. Do rights by those who have helped you, and watch God make your life for the better. Do wrong, and watch God let the Devil have a field day with you. Be grateful for the things in your life, and let no one take away from it. It is your life to live; you have to want to live the way you want your children to live one day. You can't let negative things push you in a direction that you do not want to go into. BE GRATEFUL!

Let Go!

I am a survival of Relapsing Remitting Multiple Sclerosis, and so are you. In order to be able to get through our struggle with Relapsing Remitting Multiple Sclerosis, we must continue to push through the obstacles that limit us, in order to remain positive. There are days when we become angry about being sick, and we tend to take it out on our love ones. But we must remember it is not their fault or our own. This is something that occurred and is not in our control. So we must continue to pray and talk to people who know what we are going through, and "Let Go, and Let God". Let God take the burden off our shoulders. We can't do anything about this illness other than get the best treatment in making us feel better. After all, we have a life to live, and a family who loves us very much. Thank God for family, because you only get one. Cherish every waking moment and live for God, family, friends, and yourself. Helping others to overcome or become strong in this test. God could be using you to help someone else to become as strong as you. Be an example, and live by example, so that your life can help others to overcome this obstacle we call Relapsing remitting Multiple Sclerosis. Stay true to yourself as well as others. The truth will set you free! In the book," Prayers for Good Times and Bad", states a prayer I thought is a great encouragement for you and for me; it is called:

Letting Go

Sometimes, God, I wish I could control the events in my life that cause me anxiety. Please help me to let go of my need to control things and to allow your plan for my life to unfold before me. I will trust in you, God, to show me the way.

Be Thankful!

Thank God when the pain comes and when the pain goes. Thank God when you are up, and when you are down. Thank God when you are strong, and when you are weak. Thank God for everything! Thank God when you become victorious over your illness. You are a winner over Relapsing Remitting Multiple Sclerosis. You are an overcomer! Live life as a champion; not in defeat.

Empower Others

Use your illness to empower others. Talk about it, Teach people about it, share your story with people who may be going through the same thing, and show them how to overcome it, by using your experience as a motivation. Being in denial about your illness, will only hinder your progress, and make you make wrong decisions when it comes to your healing process. God gives his strongest trials to his strongest soldiers. You'll find the strength you never thought you had, when you are stricken with a disease. Just as God was strong up on the cross, you can be strong through your circumstances. Be the bravest person you know you can be in this life. Know that this illness is only a temporary test we all must defeat. I look at Relapsing Remitting Multiple Sclerosis as another stepping stone I must climb in order to get to what God has for me in the future. I will not allow Relapsing Remitting Multiple Sclerosis to take away what I am destined to receive in the future. You should not allow it either. Don't fall every time you hit a bump in the road. Get up, dust yourself off, and keep on pushing. You will find your strength through your circumstance. Remember, God has not given up on you. Through my darkest hour, God never leaves me or forsake me. His presence comforts me, and gives me the courage to keep going no matter what my circumstances are (How to Let God Help You in Hard

Times). God's timing is not like our timing. That is why we must wait on God for our needs, and not do it for ourselves. Wait on the Lord! You can't believe he will heal you, if you don't have a relationship with Him. If you take the time to get to know him, he will show you ways to get through this obstacle if you faint not. I'm reminded of a poem from the book, "How to Let God Help You through Hard Times", which states:

We are promised that god's never early,
But neither is God ever late.
All the blessing we wish will come to us
When we learn to have faith, while we wait.
When I am lost and discouraged,
And there seems to be no hope in sight,
I turn my cares over to the God of my heart,
And His love lets my spirit take flight.

This poem really encourages me to keep fighting this battle with Relapsing Remitting Multiple Sclerosis. It should be an encouragement to you to do the same. I hope by writing this book, allow you to see your life in a different light than before. I hope it gets you out the darkness you are in, and move toward your future and the life God has for you. Take up thy cross and walk. Don't let Relapsing Remitting Multiple Sclerosis be the end of the road for you. Keep on pushing every step of the way. Don't give up on God. In the book, "How to Let God Help You through Hard Times", it states an "I Will" encouragement. It is as follows:

I WILL!

I will be strong in the face of weakness.
I will be brave in the face of fear.
I will persist in the face of failure.
I will stand again no matter how many times I fall.
I will follow my path no matter how often I lose my way.

I will live my dream no matter what obstacles stand before
me.
I will be mighty.
I will be bold.
I will be what God intended me to be.
I WILL!

In our battle with Relapsing Remitting Multiple Sclerosis, we should have an I Will spirit, simply because it lets you know that no matter what obstacle we have to face with our disease, we should not allow it to affect how we live our lives on a daily basis. We should turn our illness into a testimony. A testimony that will help others to be brave, and strive to get better. Joshua 1:9 says, have I not commanded you? Be strong and of good courage; do not be afraid, nor be dismayed, for the Lord your God is with you wherever you go". No matter what obstacle Relapsing Remitting Multiple Sclerosis puts you through this, if you continue to pray and seek him on a consistent basis. Pray for yourself, the doctors, and whatever you have to come in contact with. Have Faith! God never break his promises. God loves us in the midst of our pain, and when you feel that you are alone. Our suffering can take several things away from us, such as family, friends, health, career, and our happiness. There is one thing suffering can't take away; it can't take away the love that God has for us (Ray Pritchard, The Road Best Travelled). If everything seems to be falling to pieces, know that you have a comforter in God. God will take care of you no matter what obstacle we face. Cast your cares on Him, and watch god change your situation. I know you want to ask, why do I have so much faith in God? Though I'm battling a disease that is incurable, I believe God can heal me like he did Job in the Old Testament. Job had faith in God when he lost everything. When you go through something in life, and you know that no one in the world but God can deliver you from an incurable disease, God is who I know can heal me. He has done it before, and I know he will do it again if I only trust Him. I dedicated my life in trusting, and believing, in

God. I know that He will do what he said he's going to do. That is why I want you to get to know him for yourself. I have to admit, life has brought many painful circumstances in my life that has really caused me to waver in my faith. But, I do believe that you do have my best interests at heart, and you would never put my life in danger to a point of me forgetting who I am serving. I might not fully understand the reasons you got me going through this illness, I have choose to trust you anyway. It is a reason why I'm going through this test, but I know that you will bring me out of it. I must go through it to see where you are taking me in my future. I don't know what the future holds, but I am willing to find out if you allow me to. I have to get into my word (BIBLE) to get an understanding of what God is trying to do. He has revealed some things that I must do to get through this test. So, that is why I have dedicated my life in serving him, and going back to what he first introduce me to, and that is getting a better relationship with him. In the book, "Can We Talk? Soul stirring conversations with God by Priscilla Shirer quoted a scripture I thought is a great encouragement as well to me and those who need that strength to get through the most difficult days. It is as follows:

> "If you'll hold on to me for Dear life", says GOD,
> "I'll get you out of any trouble. I'll give you the best of care if
> you'll only get to know and trust me. Call me and
> I'll answer, be at your side in bad times;
> I'll rescue you, and then throw you a party.
> I'll give you a long life, give you a long drink of salvation!"
> Psalm 91:14-16, MSG

One thing we all can take from the scriptures and encouragements is that we are all strong individuals who know what we have to do in order to live a healthier life. We have to once again, change our mindsets, our unhealthy habits, and the people who we know does not have our best interests at heart. We need to make better choices in the things we do, because, it can damper the life we want for ourselves.

We cannot let anyone deter or make life decisions for us. We should be in control of our lives; no one should make the choices they think are right for us. After all, we are the one battling an illness, not them. Once we realize this, the better our lives, and our ability to defeat this illness. I said defeat because even though they don't have a cure, I do believe that we can one day go to the doctor, and he would say you are cured of Relapsing Remitting Multiple Sclerosis, and now you can truly live life, but with better choices. That is how strong my faith is, I believe that everyone will one day defeat this illness, if we get our lives in order. How great this would be! I know, I have strong confidence; why not? I have no other choice but to trust and believe in GOD, myself, and the doctors he allows to take care of us on a daily or yearly basis. Don't get me wrong, I am not that old, I was diagnosed with Relapsing Remitting Multiple Sclerosis at the age of thirty years old, and now I'm thirty-three years old. I am very wise for my age, I been through enough in my life to know who has brought me through several circumstances, and to lean and to depend on nobody but the GOD I serve. It doesn't take a rocket scientist to know who got you through tests you know that the doctors couldn't get you out of. That is why I am encouraging you so you do not let this illness be the end of the road for you. You must be strong and find some encouragement whether it be from the bible, family, friends, or even therapies that will help you to get through times and there will be many, that will cause you to want to give up or become depressed. Isn't your life worth living? If you do not want to live, think about the people you would be hurting who thinks you are important. Your life is not worth giving up all because you think your life is ruin because of an illness. Keep on fighting to live, I know I am not going to give up my life for anyone. I love my life, and how far I have come. I am going to fight this illness until I have no more fight in me. You should do the same thing too! Don't be left with burdens that God never intended for you to handle. Give God all your worries, stresses, all things that interrupt you living a productive life. Our burdens are too big for us to carry on our own.

Cast your cares on the Lord and he will sustain you;
He will never let the righteous fall.
Psalm 55:22

Though we are all in a trial of our own today, and the last thing you want to do is praise God. If you praise God, in the midst of your trials, you could very well help someone who is not strong as you. If you live a life like a champion, you may find out that the Lord will turn your trial into a testimony for anyone who has lost all hope in God. You could be the very person who could turn someone's life around for the better all because of how much you trust Him in your life. In the book, "Life On Purpose", says a prayer I thought is an encouragement as well. We need to recite this prayer on a daily basis in our fight with this illness. It is as follows:

Lord, forgive me for the times I've grumbled and felt sorry
for
Myself in times of trouble. I ask You to remind me that You
deserve praise through all my ups and downs. Help me to
realize how blessed I really am, and give me a thankful heart.
Thank You that my example will change the lives of others for
Your glory!

Once we realize how real God is in our lives, the better off we will be. I do not judge anyone who belief is different from mines; I do recognize that everyone is not going to believe in what I believe in, but I am speaking to those who do. Those who do not believe in what I believe in, I hope this book does not offend you. My intentions are to encourage you on a spiritual level, not to down play what you believe in. No matter what your beliefs are, God is very real in all of our lives. It all boils down to that one day we all going to get a chance to meet Him. It's easy to worship God when everything in our lives is going good. But, when things go bad, is when true worship takes place. Philip Yancey says it best: "Any relationship involves times of closeness and times of distance, and in a relationship with God, no matter how intimate, the pendulum will swing from one side to the other". That's when worship gets difficult. We must realize that God uses our circumstances to draw us closer to Him. Our circumstances are not there to punish us, but to get us where God wants us to be in the future. We all have a purpose to fulfill in life, and we must follow God's written instructions he has for us in order to get to the next level in Him. When battling with Relapsing Remitting Multiple Sclerosis, we must remember that our illness is not one we should hide from everyone. God gave us a life message to testify to others on how God brought you circumstances in your life to bring others to Him. He uses us to get his message across, so he can bring lost souls unto Him. I am very grateful that God uses me each and every day to get his message across to other people. I know that if I continue to share my story with others, that when the weak look up unto me, for the strength they have lost along the way. I have a long way to go, but I am getting there. Yes I am going through a trial right now, but that do not take away my love for God. I will serve Him until the day I die; and there is no one who can ever take that away from me. My life is a testimony, and I am going to share it with anyone who wants to listen. I hope by sharing my testimony that it don't offend those who are sick as myself, but to get you to open up more and come to terms about your illness and not to feel as if the world going to end because you are sick. It could be much worst; but God gave us a second chance to get it right with Him. So why not do it; if you can't do it for yourself, do it for those who look up to you. That is why I'm writing this book; I never thought I was going to be able to do it, but I had to be my own encouragement so that I can complete a task that I thought was impossible. When I start writing this book, I told my mom and sister and they did not believe me. I guess they thought I was not serious, but I am and look at me now, and how far I have come. This could be a start of a new adventure for me, and to the millions of people who would share in this adventure with me. I hope you enjoy it, and give to anyone who is going through a trial at this very moment. In the book, "Prayers that Avail much", states a prayer that I thought is of great importance when battling any illness. It is as follows:

> Father, in the name of Jesus, I confess Your Word
> Concerning healing. As I do this, I believe and say that Your
> Word
> Will not return to you void, but will accomplish what it says
> it will. therefore, I believe in the name of Jesus that I am
> healed, according to
> I Peter 2:24. It is written in Your Word that Jesus himself took
> our
> Infirmities and bore our sicknesses. Therefore, with great
> boldness and confidence I say on the authority of that written
> Word that I am redeemed from the curse of sickness, and I
> refuse to tolerate its symptoms. In Jesus name I pray, Amen.

Once we can come in terms with this illness, the better we are able in coping with it on a daily basis. We are to deal with this illness head on in order to handle it when it gets hard. We cannot push this illness under the rug sort of speak, because we all know that this illness is going to show up in a major way and we must be able to deal with it, when we feel that it is going to control our every aspect of our daily life. You have the power to walk in your destiny! How you choose to handle it is all up to you; the ball is in your court. You choose the direction you want to go, and let no one tell you how you should live your life. Do what is created inside you; you are a survival, and you should live your life as such. Don't live a life in defeat; live a life that is full of love, and acceptance, and not ridicule by hate, disappointment or shame. It's not your fault you have to go through this illness, think of it as God's way of preparing you for greater things. Enjoy your life to the fullest, don't let your illness damper your life and that of your friends, and family. Live a life in that your family would be proud of. Most of all live a life that you will be proud of and one day can tell your children, so they can have a role model to reference to the people that they love as well. My goal is to make you understand how you can take the necessary steps to live a much healthier life, and enjoy your life to the fullest. Appreciate the life you have now, you only get one. Don't let the world get the best of you, you get the best out of the world. If you do what you know are destine for you to do, you wouldn't have the time to form a pity party or feel down in the dumps. Do what comes natural; be true to yourself and to the people who is around you. Believe me there are people out there who looks up to you. That is why it's so important to live a life that people can look up to you for and not one that can take them on a path of destruction. Be careful how you live your life in front of people and behind closed doors. People is going to judge you no matter what, but, let them judge you of how well you live your life, and not what you do in your life. Cause in the end, it's your life, and you cannot please everyone. Do what is right, and not what people expect you to do. Don't let your adversities take over your life; yes you are going to have several issues when dealing with Relapsing Remitting Multiple Sclerosis, and you are going to have days when you feel angry, depressed, and even stressed, but, you can either move forward or you can waddle in the misery of your illness. The choice is yours; for me, I had to learn how to fight even when I didn't feel like fighting. I had to endure a lot of pain, body movements I could not stop, slurring of my speech, and problems writing. I knew that I had to go through some things in order to get to what God had for me. I knew I could not do it if I gave up or stop trying to fight. You can never win a race when you give up when trouble arises. When the trouble arises, that's when you fight even harder; you tell your illness that you are not going to let it defeat you. You are a survival, and you will fight this illness hands on and you will not give up. You have come a long way to let some illness take you out. Keep on pressing on and don't let any illness, people, or family make you feel like it is the end of the world for you. Don't get me wrong, your family is a perfect example of you feeling down in the dumps sometimes. Your family should be encouraging you, not telling you what your limits are, or what you can or cannot do. It is not there decision, it is yours. You know your limits;

and for me, I know my limits, but I choose to bust through my limits by over doing what my illness won't allow me to do. I have decided to make my body work for me, and not let my body stop me from doing what I enjoy doing. I am an over achiever, and I like to complete several goals that is going to let me make a better living for me and my children. My family does not understand me, they think I do too much; but I don't care. It's my life, and I am going to live my life to the fullest without them trying to put limitations on what I can do. In my mind, I do not have any limitations; my goal is to do all I can while I can. I am going to do just that; my family may think I am being rebellious, but I am not. I just choose to live my life how I want without the opinion of others. You should too! If we let the opinion of others hinder what we are set out to do in our lives, we are going to go nowhere. If you want to live your life, live it; don't worry about what others are going to say, they are going to talk anyway; let them talk. By them talking, should not stop you from doing you or being the person God wants you to be. You are not here to please them; you are here to please God and Him only. What others say about or to you should not matter at all. Give them something to talk about; after all, you are the one sick and already have to deal with the problems of this illness, not them. Life is too short to worry about what people say about you. They are the ones who have the problem, not you. Move on with your life, and the ones who are causing a hindrance, erase them out of your life, and replace them with people who are going to help you move forward in life, and not hate you for wanting a better life than what they are comfortable with. Sometimes, you have to think outside the box; people are not ready for change, I am ready, and I am not going to let no body get in the way of me achieving my goals. You should not either; you should be able to express yourself for the person you are, not for the person they want to mode you to be. My life has not always been peaches and cream, but I do know that I have a purpose to fulfill in this life, and I think it is for me to reach out to the many people who need that help of coming into terms with their illness as well as reach the lost souls around the world. I know my illness is a testimony for someone else, but I also know that I have a gift to encourage people. I hope that you find this book a great example of that; I hope it helps you on a more spiritual level as well as help you find out more about yourself than you could ever imagine. I am writing this book not only to help you, but to also help me as we all travel on this journey we call life. We are here for a short time anyway, why not makes the best out of the life we have here on earth before we transition into the next life. We must try the hardest to move forward in life in order to help those you most desperately need us. If you believe it or not, people do look to us for strength, why not try to be there for them. I know that we need people to help us to get through the most difficult times in our own lives, but I feel that if I could help others, I am more content. I find myself putting my needs on the back burner because I want to ensure that I could try to fulfill the needs of others. I am not a selfish person, but I want to always make people feel happy even if I am not in a good mood. To see the smile on other people faces makes me happy because I know I am doing what God is intended for me to do. I may go through a lot, but I don't let that change my attitude towards other people, whether they like me or not. I welcome all people no matter what race they are; I have a love for people, and I want people to love me as much as I love them. You don't have to get on the level of people who don't accept you; you just keep on treating them with respect, they may change their attitude. If not, keeps it moving; you don't have the time or energy to worry about how they feel about you. You have a life to live with them or without them. Remember, they have the problem, and not you. You can't please everybody, and everybody is not going to rejoice in you being blessed either. You just have to pray for them, and keep on moving into your destiny. Don't let how people treat you affect your life; cause in the end, you have earn your reward, and they have to explain themselves on judgment day. That is why it is so important to be cautious who you share your illness with; not everybody going to give you positive encouragement. There will be people who will talk negative of your illness; the people who talks negative, remove yourself from them, and find people who are going to give you positive encouragement. You already dealing with the problems that come along with Relapsing Remitting Multiple Sclerosis, you don't need people to make the situation worse than it already is. Won't the world be a much better place, if people would encourage others instead of tearing them down? My word to those who speaks negative of me is to STOP HATING! Just because people are sick does not mean we are dying, it means that God has a much better plan in the works for us. I look at my illness as a new road I must travel in order to get to a new road that is filled with more blessings and accomplishments I have to complete in order to get to the next level in my life. You should look at your life as a reward instead of a downfall; an accomplishment instead of a disappointment. Your life is a blessing from God! Relish it with love and encouragement, and stop letting the words of others stop you from achieving your dreams. If I had allowed what people say about me affect how I want to live my life, I would get nowhere in life. I don't want to live a life based on what people say; I want to live a life based on the principles of God. If you don't stand for something, you will fall for anything. Why not do what makes you feel good and not how people make you feel. Will you help me by doing what makes you feel good for once in your life? Do what makes you happy! Your happiness is what will get you through the darkest days of your life. I feel like I am on top of the world! I am a fighter that will not give up; you should feel the same way. Giving up is not an option! If you give up, it's because you have not tried your hardest; stay in the fight! Fight till there is no more fight in you. The only way to defeat this illness is to keep moving, and not to become lazy and angry. You have to be the one who defeat all odds no matter what stage you are in your illness. Look to your future, and to what is going on right now. Live life in the moment and not in the way you feel. Dismiss your feelings and keep on moving; after all, Multiple Sclerosis is all about you moving and not about you stop moving. I want to have a voice in this world; I don't want to be made silent because of a debilitating illness. Voice how you feel about anything you are going through. Don't just be like a lump on a log afraid to express your feelings. I feel a whole lot better when I get a whole lot of things off my chest. It releases a lot of tension, and stress I am bothered with on a daily basis. Don't you feel better when you release something's that are bothering you? If not, try exercising, going to a spa, or just having me time. I find that doing these entire things make me feel better and allow me to regroup my life stresses and handle them in a much better way. It won't allow me to go off on family or friends when I'm feeling my lowest. When I get away for a while, I can better deal with issues than when I am around people I feel make me angry. There is another poem that is an encouragement to anyone who needs a pick u upper so to speak. It is as follows:

Believe it,
Conceive it, take steps to
Achieve it.
Then leave the rest to
God and prepare to
Receive it!!
(Love Quotes and Sayings)

No matter how good or bad you think life is, wake up each day and be thankful for life. Someone somewhere else is fighting to survive (Jesus Still Saves, Heals, and Answers Prayer). Every time you feel like ending it all, just think about all the people who love you. Cause without the people who love you and encourage you to keep on fighting, where would you be today? There will be many days you are going to feel like you are not going to make it; but there is a God that says you can make it if you do not give up on yourself. I am not where God wants me to be yet, but I am trying. In my mind I know that I can win this race if I take the necessary steps to get to the finish line. That is what I want anyone who is destine to get well to do. Yes this is going to be a long road ahead of us, but we all can do it if we focus on what is most important to us. My journey has indeed been a long and stressful road; especially with all the changes my body goes through on a daily basis. My mood changes as my illness changes. My family thinks I'm bipolar; I am not, I just get frustrated with all the changes my body has to go through. I do not fully understand why my body wants to turn against me, but I know one thing for sure, I am not going to allow it to hold me down. You should not either; yes we are going to deal with aches and pains, but we do not have to let it take over our lives. I go through many pains and not feeling well symptoms, but I continue to do whatever I been doing with or without the pain in my body. Once you can take control of your life and do what you have to do to survive, the better your life will be. Let's get it together, and move to the next level in life. We do not have to settle for what the doctors is saying to us. We can take what they say and turn it into something positive to help someone else, or we can accept it and waddle in it or form our own pity party and waste away. The choice is yours; but, for me, I am going to fight to the end of time. I am not going to let what the doctors say to me destroy the life I have worked so hard for. You do not have to either. How do you think cancer patients feel? I look up to them so much because of the fight they have in them to get through the many obstacles they have to face as well as the radiations, medications, and the hospital stays they must endure because of the many reactions from the medications. If they can endure and keep on pushing through life as if they weren't sick, so can us. What is stopping you from living the life you once did before? What is stopping you from achieving more goals? What is making you feel ashamed of the illness you have? No one should not give up on life; life has not given up on us, so why are we so ready to give up when the going gets tough? Life is not going to be an easy task; so be ready for whatever life throws at you. The best you can do is keep jumping over pot holes that seems to want to sink us in. If you allow for what life throws at you consumes you, where would you be then? That is why it's so important for those who are sick, to never give up on life. Just because you are sick does not mean for you to act as if you are already dead. I tell my mom all the time, when she talks as if I'm already dead, that I am not dead, and don't treat me as if I'm dead already. What sick people you know want to hear that? I don't know anyone who wants to hear that. I watches commercial on television one day that has a guy talking about how he want to spend more time with his children and grandchildren because he does not have long to live. That stressed me and upset me at the same time because by me being sick, why would anyone want to see something like that? That is why I don't watch much television much because what is being said; especially when people are sick. I want to see more commercials on how or what steps a sick person are taking to prolong their life, not end it. We should not be subjected to things that make us feel like we are going to die, so why not talk as if we are already dead. NOT!! That is not my goal; my goal is to find ways to make our lives better, not frustrate us any more than we are already are. I hope this book is proven to be one that is encouraging to everyone who needs that push to get through sickness and the depressing mood it puts us all in. I hope this book is of great importance to you and others on how you can deal with any crisis in life concerning sickness. You can get through this if you stay focus and do all you can while you can. Life should be celebrated, not frustrated! Enjoy the life God has given you, and help someone else along the way. Start living your life for you and not anyone else; you are not pleasing people, you are pleasing God and yourself. Stop letting circumstances take away the life you have, and start to live life to the fullest. You only get one life, and one family, so cherish every moment that you have with them. Life is too important to let people control how you should live it. You are in control of you, and not anybody else; you choose how to live life as you did before. You should not let anything get in the way of how you should live, and accomplish any goals in life. After all, you are the champion of your life; act like you are and let's take the steps in accomplishing it. I hope this book is worth you reading it. I believe it help me as well as I am helping you to better deal with the stresses of being sick. As long as you have the support of people who love and care for you, nothing else matters. As Marvin Sapp says, "Something's you'll never get over, you just have to find ways to get through them". Getting through your circumstances is a great milestone for anyone who is sick. You just have to find ways to get through the many trials and tribulations that stops us from living life. My trials and tribulations are not like yours; we all have different ailments in our life that affects us in many ways. How we handle them is what gets us through the many problems we face on a daily basis. My illness may not be that far along as yours, but I am one who does what I need to do to get the best treatment I need to live a long life. You should be doing the same thing also. I love my life with all the problems and all; thanks for taking the time to read my book, and I hope it is one that is helpful and not a distress.